COMPLETE GUIDE TO UNDERSTANDING MASTECTOMY

Comprehensive Insights To Surgery Recovery, Breast Cancer Care, Reconstruction Options, Prevention Strategies, And Support Resources For Women's Health

KLEIN HOYLE

Disclaimer

The content in this book is based on the author's expertise and comprehension of the topic. The author has no affiliation or link with any corporation, business, or person. This book is meant to give general information and educational material only, and it should not be interpreted as professional medical advice. Always seek the advice of a skilled healthcare expert if you have any queries about medical issues or treatments. The author and publisher expressly disclaim any responsibility resulting directly or indirectly from the use or use of the information included in this book.

Table of Contents

ABOUT THIS BOOK

The "Complete Guide to Understanding Mastectomy" is an invaluable resource for anybody navigating the complications of mastectomy, providing thorough insights and assistance at every step of the process. This painstakingly prepared work provides readers with a wealth of information to help them make educated choices, prepare for surgery, and navigate the obstacles of recovery and beyond.

Chapter 1 provides the basis by explaining the core notion of mastectomy, distinguishing its many kinds, and discussing why people may choose this surgical procedure. This section ensures that readers are well-informed and prepared for what comes next by offering a comprehensive description of the operation as well as identifying possible risks and consequences.

Chapter 2 walks readers through the critical preparation period, from meetings with healthcare professionals to pre-operative testing and evaluations.

The need for mental and emotional preparation, as well as the need to arrange for post-operative care, is emphasized to ensure that patients feel supported and empowered throughout the process.

Chapter 3 focuses on Understanding Breast Cancer, providing readers with a vital understanding of the fundamentals of breast cancer, including diagnosis, staging, and treatment choices other than mastectomy. Readers are equipped to take proactive actions to protect their health after a thorough examination of early detection and preventive techniques.

Chapter 4 delves into the Decision-Making Process, which explains what variables to consider before deciding on a mastectomy, as well as how to engage in talks with healthcare providers and loved ones. This part also emphasizes the significance of personal preferences and lifestyle concerns, ensuring that people are secure in their choices.

Chapter 5 goes into the Surgical Procedure, providing a detailed description of mastectomy surgery, including incision kinds, anesthetic, and predicted results. By demystifying the surgical procedure, readers have a better knowledge and feeling of readiness.

Chapter 6 focuses on recovery and rehabilitation, guiding readers through immediate postoperative care, pain management measures, and the need for physical therapy and mental support. This section shines as a beacon of hope, providing practical skills and coping methods for navigating the obstacles of recovery with resilience.

Chapter 7 delves into Potential issues, providing readers with the information they need to recognize frequent post-mastectomy issues and develop preventative and treatment methods. This segment promotes a feeling of agency and preparation by teaching people when to seek medical assistance and how to grasp the long-term consequences.

Chapter 8 discusses breast reconstruction options, including an overview of techniques, eligibility criteria, and related risks and benefits. This section ensures that people are well-informed while contemplating reconstruction, allowing them to make choices based on their requirements and preferences.

Chapter 9 focuses on life after mastectomy, guiding readers through the process of adapting to physical changes, negotiating psychological and emotional effects, and accessing support networks and resources. This part prepares people to face life after mastectomy with confidence and grace by encouraging resilience and self-acceptance.

Chapter 10, Moving Forward, is a source of inspiration, including advice on follow-up treatment, healthy lifestyle choices, activism, and awareness campaigns. This part, which focuses on empowerment and community, invites readers to use their experiences to inspire others and influence good change.

In summary, the "Complete Guide to Understanding Mastectomy" goes beyond the scope of a basic informative resource, functioning as a constant companion and inspiring people to negotiate the complications of mastectomy with bravery, resilience, and everlasting optimism.

CHAPTER 1

What Is A Mastectomy?

Definition And Types Of Mastectomy

A mastectomy is a surgical surgery that removes one or both breasts. It is widely used to treat breast cancer, but it may also be used as a prophylactic measure in situations where there is a significant chance of getting breast cancer.

Mastectomy is classified into various forms, with each removing a different amount of breast tissue. The most popular kinds are:

1. **Total mastectomy:** Also known as simple mastectomy, this procedure removes the whole breast, including the nipple and areola, but does not usually remove the lymph nodes under the arm.

2. Modified radical mastectomy: This treatment removes the whole breast, including the nipple and areola, as well as the lymph nodes in the armpit.

3. Radical mastectomy is a less common treatment that involves removing the whole breast, including the nipple and areola, as well as the underlying chest muscles and lymph nodes. It is often reserved for very advanced instances of breast cancer.

4. Double mastectomy (bilateral mastectomy): This procedure includes the removal of both breasts, either as a therapy for breast cancer in both breasts or as a prophylactic step in instances where there is a significant risk of acquiring breast cancer later.

The kind of mastectomy advised will be determined by the size and location of the tumor, the stage of breast cancer, as well as the patient's general health and preferences.

Reasons For Getting A Mastectomy

Mastectomy is performed for a variety of reasons, the most common of which are to cure or prevent breast cancer. Some frequent explanations are:

1. Breast cancer therapy may include a mastectomy, especially if the tumor is big or there are several cancers in the breast. It may also be indicated if the malignancy has progressed to the chest muscles or adjacent lymph nodes.

2. **Prophylactic mastectomy:** In situations where there is a high chance of acquiring breast cancer, such as with certain genetic abnormalities (e.g., BRCA1 or BRCA2), a prophylactic mastectomy may be indicated to lower the risk of developing the illness. This is often done prophylactically in persons who have a family history of breast cancer or who have tested positive for certain genetic abnormalities.

3. Risk reduction: Even in the absence of a cancer diagnosis, some people may opt to have a mastectomy to lower their chances of getting breast cancer, especially if they have a significant family history of the illness or other risk factors.

4. Other benign (non-cancerous) breast disorders that may be treated with a mastectomy include severe fibrocystic alterations, recurring infections, and big tumors that cause pain or discomfort.

5. Cosmetic considerations: In certain situations, people may choose mastectomy as part of their treatment plan for cosmetic reasons, such as achieving symmetry if only one breast is damaged by cancer or improving the outcome of breast reconstruction surgery.

The choice to get a mastectomy is very personal and should be taken in conjunction with a healthcare physician after carefully weighing the risks and benefits.

Overview Of The Surgical Procedure

Patients often undergo a battery of preoperative assessments before mastectomy, including imaging tests (such as mammography or MRI) and, in some cases, a biopsy to confirm the presence of cancer cells.

On the day of surgery, patients are frequently given general anesthesia to keep them comfortable and pain-free during the operation. The surgeon next creates an incision in the breast using preset marks to guarantee optimum tissue removal.

Depending on the kind of mastectomy done, the surgeon will remove varied amounts of breast tissue, such as the complete breast or a part of it. If lymph nodes are being removed, the surgeon will gently dissect and remove them from the armpit.

After the appropriate tissue has been removed, the surgeon will carefully seal the wounds with sutures or surgical staples. In rare circumstances, drains may be inserted to remove excess fluid from the surgical site and facilitate recovery.

Following surgery, patients are carefully observed in the recovery area before being transported to a hospital room or released home, depending on the severity of the operation and their general health. Pain management and wound care instructions will be given, and follow-up consultations will be planned to evaluate progress and discuss any further treatment choices, such as chemotherapy or radiation therapy.

Possible Hazards And Complications

Mastectomy, like any other surgical treatment, has risks and consequences. Some of them may include:

1. **Bleeding:** Excessive bleeding during or after surgery is conceivable, although it is uncommon and normally controlled by the surgical team.

2. Infection: There is a possibility of developing an infection at the surgery site, which may need antibiotics or other medical care.

3. Changes in feeling: After a mastectomy, some people may suffer temporary or permanent changes in sensation or numbness in their chest, breast, or surrounding regions.

4. Lymphedema: The removal of lymph nodes may interrupt the normal outflow of lymphatic fluid, causing swelling and pain in the arm on the afflicted side.

5. Seroma: Fluid collection in the surgical site (seroma) is a frequent consequence after mastectomy, although it is typically treatable with drainage or aspiration.

6. Wound healing issues: Delayed wound healing or wound breakdown may occur, especially in those who smoke, have diabetes, or have other underlying medical factors that might impair healing.

7. Cosmetic changes: A mastectomy may have a substantial influence on a person's body image and self-esteem, especially if breast reconstruction is not sought or difficulties occur during the reconstruction procedure.

Individuals seeking mastectomy should discuss the possible risks and consequences with their healthcare professional and measure them against the advantages of the treatment. Furthermore, according to postoperative care instructions attending follow-up visits may reduce the risk of problems while promoting optimum recovery.

CHAPTER 2

Preparing For Mastectomy

Consultation With Healthcare Providers

Before having a mastectomy, you should have extensive discussions with your healthcare experts. These meetings usually include conversations with your surgeon, oncologist, and other medical specialists engaged in your treatment. During these sessions, you will be able to ask questions, voice your concerns, and learn about the process.

Your surgeon will discuss the sort of mastectomy that is most suited to your condition, such as a whole mastectomy, a partial mastectomy, or a radical mastectomy. They will explain why they suggest each alternative, as well as the possible risks and advantages.

Furthermore, your healthcare team will examine your medical history, including any past operations, medical issues, and drugs you are presently using. This information allows them to personalize the treatment strategy to your specific requirements while minimizing possible issues during and after the surgery.

Pre-Operative Tests And Assessments

Before having mastectomy surgery, you will go through various pre-operative examinations and evaluations to ensure you are physically prepared for the treatment. These tests may include blood tests, imaging scans (e.g., mammograms or MRI scans), and electrocardiograms (ECGs) to assess heart function.

These tests assist your healthcare team in determining any underlying medical issues that may impact your operation or recovery. For example, if you have heart problems or diabetes, your doctor may take extra steps to keep you safe throughout the surgery.

In rare situations, a breast biopsy may be performed to confirm the existence of cancer or other abnormalities. This biopsy serves to guide the surgical approach and ensures that the correct portions of tissue are removed during the mastectomy.

Mental And Emotional Preparation

Preparing for mastectomy surgery entails both physical and mental preparation. Facing the idea of breast surgery may cause a wide variety of feelings, including dread, worry, grief, and uncertainty.

During this period, it is critical to seek assistance from family, friends, and healthcare experts. Many hospitals provide counseling services or support groups exclusively for those undergoing breast cancer surgery. These websites may give helpful emotional support as well as practical assistance for dealing with the next obstacles.

It is also beneficial to educate yourself about the process and what to anticipate before and after surgery. Understanding the process may assist in reducing worry and allow you to make educated choices regarding your treatment.

Arrangements For Postoperative Care

In addition to preparing for the operation, it is critical to plan for post-operative care to ensure a smooth recovery. This might include scheduling help from friends or family members with domestic tasks, childcare, or transportation to follow-up visits.

Your healthcare team will provide you with detailed instructions for post-operative care, such as wound care, pain management, and activity limitations. It is essential to follow these recommendations precisely to reduce the risk of problems and enhance recovery.

You may also need to arrange for any medical equipment or supplies, such as compression garments or drainage tubes, to help with your recuperation at home. Your healthcare team can assist you with these difficulties and ensure you have all you need for a good recovery.

Taking these actions to prepare for mastectomy surgery will help assure the best possible result while also supporting your physical, mental, and emotional well-being during the procedure.

CHAPTER 3

Understanding Breast Cancer

Basics Of Breast Cancer

Breast cancer starts in the cells of the breast. The two most prevalent kinds are ductal carcinoma, which develops in duct cells, and lobular carcinoma, which begins in lobules. Understanding the architecture of the breast helps us understand how cancer develops. The breast is made up of lobules (milk-producing glands), ducts (small tubes that transport milk to the nipple), fatty and connective tissue, blood arteries, and lymph nodes.

Breast cancer develops when cells in the breast continue to proliferate uncontrolled. These cells often form a tumor, which may be visible on X-rays or felt as a bump. It is crucial to understand that not all tumors are malignant.

Benign (non-cancerous) breast tumors are abnormal growths that do not extend beyond the breast and are not life-threatening.

Breast cancer has many risk factors, including genetic abnormalities (such as BRCA1 and BRCA2), age, family history, personal health history, and specific lifestyle choices. However, having one or more risk factors does not guarantee that a person will get breast cancer. It simply implies a greater chance compared to the overall population.

Diagnoses And Staging

Diagnosis

Breast cancer is often diagnosed when a person discovers a lump or irregularity in their breast. However, many instances are discovered early on by standard mammography screening. Once an anomaly is identified, various measures are required to determine the existence and kind of breast cancer:

1. Physical examination: The doctor checks the breasts and surrounding regions for lumps or anomalies.

2. Mammograms, ultrasounds, and magnetic resonance imaging (MRI) all assist in providing detailed images of the breast. These tests may detect the existence of a tumor and offer details about its size and location.

3. Biopsy: If imaging studies show a questionable region, a biopsy is conducted. A biopsy involves removing a sample of breast tissue and examining it under a microscope for cancer cells. Biopsies come in three types: fine-needle aspiration, core needle biopsy, and surgical biopsy.

Staging

Staging indicates the degree of cancer throughout the body, which is critical for deciding treatment choices and prognosis. Breast cancer staging depends on several factors:

1. Tumor Size (T): The size of the tumor within the breast.

2. Node Involvement (N) indicates if cancer has spread to surrounding lymph nodes.

3. Metastasis (M) indicates if cancer has migrated to other regions of the body.

Stages vary from zero to four, with higher numbers signifying more advanced cancer:

• Stage 0 is non-invasive malignancy (ductal carcinoma in situ).

• Stage I cancer is small and invasive, with limited or no lymph node involvement.

• Stage II cancers are larger and involve more lymph nodes.

• Stage III has more lymph nodes and bigger tumors.

• Metastatic breast cancer in Stage IV refers to cancer that has spread to distant organs.

Treatment Options Beyond Mastectomy

Chemotherapy

Chemotherapy employs chemicals to eliminate cancer cells. It may be used before surgery (neoadjuvant) to reduce tumors or after surgery (adjuvant) to eradicate any leftover cancer cells. Chemotherapy is also used to treat metastatic breast cancer. The therapy consists of medication delivery in cycles separated by rest intervals to enable the body to recuperate. Fatigue, hair loss, nausea, and an increase in infection risk are all possible side effects.

Radiation Therapy

Radiation treatment employs high-energy waves to target and kill cancer cells. It is often used after surgery to eliminate any leftover cancer cells in the breast, chest wall, or axilla (underarm region). The most frequent form is external beam radiation, which is generated by a machine and directed to the afflicted region. Another method is brachytherapy, which involves implanting radioactive seeds in the breast near the tumor location.

Hormone Therapy

Hormone therapy is used to treat malignancies that are hormone receptor-positive. These tumors develop in response to hormones such as estrogen and progesterone. Treatments include pharmaceuticals that prevent hormones from binding to cancer cells (e.g., tamoxifen) and drugs that suppress hormone levels in the body (e.g., aromatase inhibitors). Hormone treatment may be administered before or after surgery to reduce the likelihood of recurrence.

Targeted therapy

Targeted treatments target particular chemicals involved in cancer cell proliferation and survival. Examples include HER2 inhibitors (such as trastuzumab) for HER2-positive breast cancer and

CDK4/6 inhibitors for specific forms of metastatic breast cancer. These medicines are often used in conjunction with other therapies to increase efficacy, and they might cause adverse effects such as cardiac problems or exhaustion.

Immunotherapy

Immunotherapy allows the immune system to detect and fight cancer cells. While it is still relatively new in the treatment of breast cancer, it shows promise, especially in triple-negative cases. Immune checkpoint inhibitors are the most prevalent kind, which serves to release the immune system's brakes, allowing it to combat cancer more effectively.

Importance Of Early Detection And Prevention

Early detection

Early identification of breast cancer significantly improves the likelihood of effective treatment and survival.

Key strategies for early detection include:

• Regular self-examination allows people to get comfortable with their breasts and detect any changes.

• Clinician-performed breast examinations are advised every 1-3 years for women aged 20-39 and yearly for those 40+.

• Mammography is the most effective screening method to identify breast cancer early. Women aged 40 and over should get mammograms every 1-2 years, depending on their risk factors and doctor's recommendations.

Prevention

While not all breast cancers are preventable, several steps may lower the risk:

• A healthy lifestyle includes maintaining a healthy weight, eating a balanced diet, limiting alcohol use, and exercising frequently to reduce risk.

• Tobacco use is connected to several cancers, including breast cancer. Avoid smoking.

• For postmenopausal hormone treatment, utilize the lowest effective dosage for the shortest time feasible.

• Genetic Testing and Preventive Surgery: For individuals with a significant family history or genetic susceptibility (BRCA mutations), genetic testing may inform preventive procedures like prophylactic mastectomy or oophorectomy.

Understanding these elements of breast cancer allows people to make proactive efforts to monitor their health and make educated choices regarding their treatment.

CHAPTER 4

Decision-Making Process

Factors To Consider Before Deciding On A Mastectomy

The choice to have a mastectomy is an important and personal one, affected by a variety of medical, emotional, and practical considerations. Understanding these characteristics may help people make educated decisions that are consistent with their health requirements and personal beliefs.

Medical Considerations

1. Diagnosis and Stage of Cancer: The kind and stage of breast cancer are important in evaluating whether a mastectomy is required. For example, more severe or advanced malignancies may need a mastectomy over alternative therapies, such as a lumpectomy.

2. Genetic Factors: People who have BRCA1 or BRCA2 gene mutations are more likely to develop breast cancer and may choose preventive mastectomy to lower their risk.

3. Previous Treatments: Previous surgeries, radiation, or chemotherapy may affect the feasibility and need for a mastectomy.

4. Overall Health: The existence of additional medical problems, as well as general health, might have an impact on surgical choices. Patients in excellent health may have more choices and have fewer difficulties.

Emotional and Psychological Considerations

1. Losing one or both breasts may have a profound influence on body image and self-esteem. Understanding these consequences and contemplating post-surgical reconstructive possibilities is critical.

2. Fear and Anxiety: Concerns about cancer recurrence may have a significant impact on decision-making.

Some people may feel more comfortable undergoing a mastectomy to remove as much tissue as feasible.

3. Mental Health Support: Having access to mental health specialists may assist address the psychological effects and guide people through the decision-making process.

Practical considerations

1. Healing Time and Impact on Daily Life: The healing period after a mastectomy may be lengthy, necessitating time off work and assistance with daily tasks. It is critical to prepare for this and understand the logistical implications.

2. Financial Implications: The expense of surgery, follow-up therapies, and possible reconstruction should be addressed. Insurance coverage and out-of-pocket payments should be thoroughly examined.

3. Support System: Having a robust support system in place, including family, friends, and community resources, is critical for postoperative healing and emotional support.

Discussions With The Healthcare Team And Loved Ones

An open and comprehensive discussion with both healthcare experts and loved ones is essential for making an educated choice regarding a mastectomy.

Consult the Healthcare Team.

1. Medical Expertise: Surgeons, oncologists, and plastic surgeons may give valuable insights about the medical needs, risks, and advantages of mastectomy. They can discuss alternative therapies and what to anticipate after surgery.

2. Personalized advice: Each patient's condition is unique, and healthcare practitioners may give tailored advice based on medical history, current health, and personal circumstances.

3. Clarifying Doubts: It is important to ask questions and explain any concerns concerning the surgery, recuperation, and long-term prospects. This involves recognizing the possibility of reconstruction and other post-surgery choices.

Involving Loved Ones

1. Emotional Support: Talking about the choice with family and close friends gives emotional support and helps in the psychological management of the decision.

2. Practical Support: Family members may help with logistical preparation, such as organizing care throughout rehabilitation and handling domestic tasks.

3. Shared Decision-Making: Involving loved ones in the decision-making process ensures that the patient's support network is prepared and in sync with the patient's decisions, promoting a supportive atmosphere.

Personal Preferences And Lifestyle Considerations

Personal tastes and lifestyle concerns influence the choice to get a mastectomy. Understanding how these factors influence decision-making may assist people in making decisions that are most appropriate for their lives and ideals.

Lifestyle Factors

1. Activity Level: Active persons may be worried about how surgery and recuperation may affect their ability to participate in physical activities. Discussing these concerns with healthcare personnel may help you create realistic goals and prepare for recovery.

2. Work and Career: Consider the necessity for time off from work as well as the influence on your career. Some employees may need to work with their employers to take prolonged leave or make modifications while recovering.

3. Individuals with caring duties, whether for youngsters or elderly family members, must arrange for support throughout their rehabilitation.

Personal Preferences

1. Aesthetic Preferences: The desire for breast reconstruction, the kind of reconstruction, and the decision to wear prostheses after surgery are all very personal choices that affect body image and self-confidence.

2. Risk Tolerance: Everyone's risk tolerance is different. Some people want intensive therapy to reduce the risk of recurrence, while others prefer less intrusive choices to maintain their existing quality of life.

3. Quality of life: The possible influence on long-term health, comfort, and emotional well-being is an important consideration. Individuals must balance the advantages of surgery with the possible changes in their everyday life.

Resources For More Information And Support

Access to credible information and support networks is critical in making an educated choice regarding mastectomy. There are many services accessible to provide direction, information, and emotional support.

Educational Resources

1. Online Medical Databases: Websites such as PubMed, the National Cancer Institute, and the American Cancer Society provide comprehensive, peer-reviewed information about breast cancer therapies and mastectomy.

2. Publications and Guides: Many publications authored by medical experts and survivors give in-depth insights into the mastectomy decision-making process.

3. Healthcare Provider Materials: Many clinics and hospitals provide pamphlets, websites, and seminars to help people understand their choices.

Support Networks

1. Support Groups: Local and online support groups may provide emotional support and practical guidance from others who have gone through similar situations.

2. Counseling Services: Having access to expert counselors, such as oncology social workers and psychologists, may assist manage the emotional and psychological consequences of the choice.

3. Community Resources: Many localities have breast cancer awareness organizations, patient advocacy groups, and non-profits that may help and support people.

Personalized Assistance

1. Patient Navigators: Some healthcare systems include patient navigators that may help with scheduling, locating resources, and answering questions throughout the treatment process.

2. Peer Mentorship Programs: Programs that link patients with survivors of mastectomies may provide crucial firsthand information and support.

Individuals may make well-informed choices about obtaining a mastectomy by carefully examining these considerations, having in-depth talks with healthcare experts and loved ones, and using available resources.

CHAPTER 5

Surgical Procedures

A Step-By-Step Overview Of Mastectomy Surgery

Mastectomy surgery is an important step in the treatment of breast cancer that involves the removal of breast tissue. The process usually starts with the patient being given an anesthetic to keep them comfortable and pain-free during the operation. After the anesthetic has taken effect, the surgeon makes an incision in the skin to expose the breast tissue underneath.

The kind of incision used is determined by several criteria, including the tumor's size and location, as well as the patient's preferences. Incisions such as the radial scar, periareolar, and inframammary are common. Each incision has benefits and may provide distinct cosmetic results.

After making the incision, the surgeon gently removes the breast tissue, being sure to remove any malignant cells. In certain circumstances, the surgeon may additionally remove adjacent lymph nodes to determine the spread of malignancy. After the appropriate tissue has been removed, the wound is closed with sutures or surgical staples.

Throughout the treatment, the patient's vital signs are carefully checked to guarantee their safety and well-being. The length of the operation varies according to the size of the mastectomy and any other treatments done. However, most mastectomy operations last a few hours.

Different Types Of Incisions And Techniques

Mastectomy surgery uses a variety of incisions and procedures, each with its own set of pros and disadvantages. One popular procedure is skin-sparing mastectomy, which removes breast tissue while leaving the skin envelope intact. This method may lead to a more natural-looking breast reconstruction.

Another approach is the nipple-sparing mastectomy, which removes breast tissue while leaving the nipple and areola intact. This method is appropriate for individuals with tiny tumors positioned distant from the nipple.

In terms of incisions, the radial scar incision surrounds the areola, while the periareolar incision runs along its edge. The inframammary incision is done along the fold under the breasts. Each incision has benefits and may provide distinct cosmetic results.

Anesthesia And Monitoring During Surgery

Anesthesia is given before mastectomy surgery to keep the patient pain-free and comfortable during the treatment. The kind of anesthetic used may vary according to the patient's health and preferences. General anesthesia is routinely utilized, which renders the patient unconscious during surgery.

The anesthesia team continuously monitors the patient's vital signs during operation, including heart rate, blood pressure, and oxygen levels. This continual monitoring ensures the patient's safety and well-being during the treatment.

Duration And Expected Results

The length of mastectomy surgery varies based on several variables, including the degree of the mastectomy, the patient's general health, and any extra treatments undertaken. Mastectomy surgery typically lasts a few hours.

Patients who have had mastectomy surgery may anticipate some soreness and edema in the treated region. However, this usually resolves itself with time, and pain medicines are provided to alleviate any discomfort. Depending on the kind of mastectomy done, patients may choose breast reconstruction to restore the look of their breasts.

Overall, mastectomy surgery is an important step in the treatment of breast cancer, and the predicted results vary depending on the person. However, with careful care and follow-up, many people may recover and improve their quality of life after mastectomy surgery.

CHAPTER 6

Recovery And Rehabilitation

Immediate Postoperative Care At The Hospital

Following a mastectomy, the first phase of healing occurs in the hospital. This stage is crucial for ensuring that the body begins to recover correctly and that any urgent difficulties are handled as soon as possible.

Monitoring And Initial Assessment

After the procedure, patients are brought to a recovery room and carefully observed by healthcare experts. Vital indicators such as heart rate, blood pressure, and oxygen levels are regularly monitored to guarantee stability. The surgical site is periodically checked for symptoms of excessive bleeding or infection.

Pain Management

Effective pain management is a top goal in the early postoperative period. Patients are often given pain drugs via an intravenous (IV) line at first, and subsequently switched to oral meds when their condition improves. Pain levels are routinely measured using a pain scale, and medication doses are changed as needed to keep the patient comfortable.

Drain Management

Surgical drains are often used during mastectomy to remove excess fluid from the surgical site. These drains are generally tiny tubes attached to fluid-collecting bulbs. Nurses will show how to empty and quantify the fluid from these drains, and patients will be given information on how to care for them at home.

Mobility And Early Exercises

Early mobilization is recommended to improve circulation and avoid issues like blood clots. Nurses may assist patients in sitting up and walking a short distance. Simple arm exercises are provided to keep shoulders mobile and avoid stiffness.

Diet & Nutrition

Patients may be given clear liquids at first, followed by normal food if tolerated. A well-balanced diet high in proteins, vitamins, and minerals is advised for optimal recovery. Hospital personnel may issue nutritional suggestions for patients to follow while recovering.

Discharge Planning

Before being discharged, patients are given extensive instructions on how to care for their surgery site and drains, manage pain, identify indicators of infection or problems, and follow up with their surgeon.

Plans for home care or outpatient sessions with a physical therapist may also be established.

Managing Pain And Discomfort

Effective pain and discomfort treatment is critical for facilitating healing and improving the quality of life after a mastectomy. Several techniques may be used to address these symptoms.

Medication

Opioids, nonsteroidal anti-inflammatory medicines (NSAIDs), and acetaminophen are all popular pain relievers. The kind and dose are determined by the patient's medical history and the degree of their discomfort. Before making any adjustments, follow the specified regimen and talk with your healthcare professional.

Nonmedical Pain Relief

In addition to medicine, a variety of non-medical treatments may be used to relieve pain and discomfort. This includes:

• Cold packs may help decrease swelling and discomfort in the surgery region.

• Warm compresses may help relax muscles and relieve pain once swelling has subsided.

• Deep breathing, meditation, and guided imagery are effective relaxation techniques that may lessen pain perception.

• Massage therapy helps reduce muscular tension, increase circulation, and alleviate discomfort in the shoulders and back.

Positioning & Support

Proper placement may greatly alleviate discomfort. Using additional pillows to support the arms and upper body when resting or sleeping helps reduce tension on the surgery site. Special post-mastectomy bras or camisoles with built-in support and soft padding may also make you feel more comfortable.

Physical Therapy And Exercises

Physical therapy and exercise are essential in the post-mastectomy rehabilitation phase, as they assist in recovering mobility, strength, and function.

Initial Exercises

Gentle exercises are advised in the first few weeks after surgery to keep the shoulder and arm mobile. This includes:

• To do the Pendulum Exercise, lean forward slightly and allow the arm on the surgery side to hang down. Swing the arm gently in tiny circles.

· Wall Climbing: Face a wall and use your fingers to "climb" as far as you can. Hold the posture for a few seconds before gently sliding the hand down.

Progressive Exercises

As recovery continues, more difficult exercises may be introduced to develop strength and flexibility.

• To do arm lifts, lie on your back and bend your knees. Hold a tiny weight in your surgical hand. Slowly raise the arm straight up to the ceiling and then drop it back down.

• Shoulder Blade Squeeze: Sit or stand with arms at sides. Squeeze the shoulder blades together for a few seconds, then release.

Formal Physical Therapy

A physical therapist may create individualized workout routines and hands-on treatments to address particular conditions including scar tissue accumulation, lymphedema, and muscular weakness. They may also teach suitable strategies for doing regular tasks without strain or harm.

Emotional Support And Coping Strategies

Recovery following a mastectomy is both physical and emotional. Coping with physical changes and the effects on mental health need strong emotional support and good coping mechanisms.

Professional Support

Therapists, counselors, and support groups provide patients with a secure area to vent their emotions, anxieties, and concerns. Anxiety, sadness, and body image concerns may be managed with professional treatment. Support groups allow you to connect with people who have had similar experiences, offering mutual support and understanding.

Family And Friends

Family and friends' support is crucial throughout the rehabilitation process. Open conversation about wants and emotions may build relationships and give much-needed emotional support. Loved ones may help with everyday duties, attend appointments, and provide a listening ear.

Meditation And Relaxation Techniques

Mindfulness, meditation, and yoga are all practices that may help you relax and feel better emotionally. These approaches assist people in being present, managing their thoughts and emotions, and finding inner peace during the trials of rehabilitation.

Engaging In Hobbies And Activities

Engaging in fun activities and hobbies may create a feeling of normality while also distracting from physical pain. Maintaining an active and meaningful lifestyle, whether via reading, crafts, gardening, or other activities, is beneficial to mental wellness.

Self-Compassion And Positive Affirmations

Self-compassion is being gentle to oneself and understanding that rehabilitation is a slow process. Positive affirmations may boost self-esteem and promote a positive attitude. Celebrating little accomplishments and appreciating achievements, no matter how tiny, may increase morale and motivation.

Recovery following a mastectomy is a multidimensional process that requires both physical and emotional care. Individuals may traverse this road more comfortably and confidently if they understand the many parts of post-operative care, pain management, physical therapy, and emotional support.

CHAPTER 7

Potential Complications

Common Complications Following Mastectomy

While mastectomy is an important technique in the treatment of breast cancer, it is not without risks. Understanding these problems is critical for patients and caregivers seeking effective post-operative care and treatment.

The most frequent complication is discomfort. It is typical to feel pain and discomfort after mastectomy surgery. This discomfort may vary from minor to severe, depending on the individual's pain tolerance and the scope of the operation. Medication, physical therapy, and relaxation methods may all assist in relieving pain.

Seroma development, or swelling and fluid collection, is another typical side effect after mastectomy. Seromas may produce noticeable swelling and pain in the chest. To avoid excessive fluid accumulation, surgeons often insert drains after surgery to eliminate excess fluid. Proper drainage treatment and monitoring are required to avoid problems related to seromas.

Infection is yet another possible consequence. Surgical wounds are prone to infection, and mastectomy is no exception. Infection symptoms include redness, warmth, swelling, and increasing discomfort at the surgery site. To avoid future problems, seek medical assistance as soon as symptoms of infection appear.

Lymphedema is a long-term problem that may develop after mastectomy, especially if lymph nodes are removed during surgery. Lymphedema occurs when lymph fluid accumulates, producing swelling and pain in the afflicted arm or chest region. Physical therapy, compression garments, and lifestyle changes are often prescribed to treat lymphedema and enhance quality of life.

Strategies For Prevention And Management

Preventing problems after mastectomy requires a proactive effort from patients and healthcare professionals. Proper pre-operative preparation, such as improving general health and addressing possible risks with the surgical team, may help reduce the probability of problems.

During surgery, procedures such as precise wound closure and prophylactic antibiotic usage may help to limit the risk of infection. Surgeons may also use sophisticated surgical procedures, such as sentinel lymph node biopsy, to lessen the effect on lymphatic outflow and the risk of lymphedema.

Post-operative care is critical for minimizing problems and encouraging recovery. Following surgical instructions for drain care, wound care, and activity limitations is critical for reducing the risk of infection, seroma development, and other problems.

Patients should also be proactive in treating their pain and suffering by using medicine, physical therapy, and relaxation methods. Open contact with healthcare practitioners is critical if issues emerge, allowing for timely intervention and treatment.

When To Seek Medical Attention?

While some soreness and swelling are normal after mastectomy, some signs and symptoms need prompt medical treatment. This includes:

• Pain that persists or worsens despite medicines.

• Excessive edema, redness, warmth, or discharge at the surgery site.

• Infection symptoms include fever, chills, and flu-like symptoms.

• Difficulty breathing or chest discomfort.

Notifying healthcare professionals of any concerned symptoms early enables appropriate diagnosis and management, lowering the risk of complications and supporting optimum recovery.

Long-Term Effects And Adjustments

Beyond the immediate post-operative time, mastectomy may have long-term consequences and need lifestyle changes. Lymphedema, for example, may last eternally, necessitating continual care techniques such as compression garments and physical therapy.

Emotional and psychological adaptations are also prevalent after mastectomy, since patients may experience changes in body image and self-esteem. Breast cancer survivors may benefit greatly from support groups, therapy, and services during this time of transition.

Furthermore, constant follow-up treatment and monitoring are required to detect any symptoms of recurrence or new developments. Periodic imaging scans and physical exams are often recommended by healthcare practitioners to guarantee early identification and, if necessary, quick action.

Patients may confidently and resiliently traverse the post-mastectomy path by identifying possible risks, applying preventative techniques, knowing when to seek medical assistance, and making long-term modifications.

CHAPTER 8

Breast Reconstruction Options

Overview Of Breast Reconstruction Procedures

Breast reconstruction is a surgical treatment that restores the form and appearance of the breasts after a mastectomy or lumpectomy. Breast reconstruction may be classified into numerous forms, each with its own set of treatments and results. The two major types of reconstruction are implant-based reconstruction and autologous (or flap) reconstruction.

Implant-Based Reconstruction: This technique includes inserting a breast implant, either saline or silicone, to restore the breast mound. The treatment normally begins with the insertion of a tissue expander behind the chest muscle, which is progressively filled with saline over a period of weeks or months.

Once the skin and muscle have extended enough, the expander is replaced with a permanent implant.

Autologous (Flap) Reconstruction: This procedure reconstructs the breast using the patient's tissue obtained from another region of the body, such as the belly, back, thigh, or buttocks. The TRAM (transverse rectus abdominis muscle) flap, DIEP (deep inferior epigastric perforator) flap, and latissimus dorsi flap are among the most often used flap operations. These treatments are more difficult and require a longer recovery time, but they often result in a more natural feel and look.

Mix Procedures: Some patients may choose to use a mix of implants and flap methods to get the desired outcome. This technique may enhance volume and create a more natural shape.

Timing And Eligibility For Reconstruction

The time of breast reconstruction is crucial and may be divided into two categories: immediate reconstruction and delayed reconstruction.

Immediate Reconstruction: This takes place in the same procedure as the mastectomy. The biggest advantage is that it decreases the number of procedures and provides the psychological benefit of waking up with a restored breast. However, rapid reconstruction may not be appropriate for many patients, particularly those who need further cancer therapies, such as radiation therapy, which may influence healing and the overall esthetic result.

Delayed Reconstruction: This is done many months or even years after the original mastectomy. Delayed reconstruction may be indicated for individuals who need post-mastectomy radiotherapy or who are not suitable for quick reconstruction owing to other medical issues or personal preferences. This permits the patient to finish their cancer therapy and concentrate on recuperation before having further surgery.

Candidacy for Reconstruction: Not all patients are suitable for all types of breast reconstruction. Overall health, body type, cancer treatment strategy, and personal preferences all have an impact on eligibility. Patients with specific health concerns, such as uncontrolled diabetes or excessive smoking, may be at a greater risk of complications and should address these issues before having reconstruction.

Risks And Benefits Of Reconstruction

Breast reconstruction, like any major surgery, has possible dangers and advantages that the patient must carefully consider in cooperation with their medical team.

Risks:

• Surgical site infection is a danger associated with any operation. This may need antibiotics or extra surgery.

• \ Bleeding and hematoma: The surgical region may accumulate blood or fluid, which requires drainage.

• Implant Complications: Implants may burst, deflate, or induce capsular contracture, leading to further procedures.

• Flap Failure: Autologous reconstruction might result in partial or full flap loss if the transplanted tissue does not survive.

• Scarring: Reconstructive operations may cause varying degrees of scarring.

Benefits:

• Reconstruction may restore the natural look of the breast, leading to improved self-esteem and body image.

• Achieving breast symmetry improves garment fit and physical equilibrium.

• Emotional and psychological benefits: Reconstruction may provide closure and promote emotional well-being for women who have completed their cancer treatment.

Alternative Options For Breast Symmetry

There are various other techniques for achieving breast symmetry for people who do not want to have breast reconstruction or are not eligible for surgery.

External prostheses are silicone breast shapes that may be worn within a bra to provide the impression of a real breast. They come in a variety of forms, sizes, and skin tones, and may be tailored to complement the remaining breast.

Custom-made prostheses are molded to the individual's chest wall, resulting in a very realistic look and comfortable wear.

Adhesive Breast Forms: These are intended to cling directly to the chest wall, providing a more secure and natural appearance without the need for a specialist bra.

 Specialized clothes and swimwear with built-in pockets may securely store prostheses, providing a diverse variety of design alternatives for people who do not choose to undergo reconstruction.

Choosing the ideal alternative for breast symmetry is a very personal decision that takes into account a variety of criteria such as the patient's lifestyle, comfort level, and desired cosmetic result. Consulting with a healthcare expert may help you make an educated decision that is tailored to your specific requirements and preferences.

CHAPTER 9

Life Following Mastectomy

Adapting To Physical Changes And Limitations

Adjusting to physical changes and possible limits after a mastectomy may be an important component of the recovery process. Initially, you may feel discomfort or agony while your body recovers from surgery. Your healthcare staff will advise you on how to manage any post-operative pain and detail the rehabilitation process. It is essential to closely follow their directions to enhance healing and limit the danger of problems.

One of the most obvious physical changes is the disappearance of one or both breasts. This alteration might have an impact on your posture, balance, and general body image. Many people discover that using customized bras or prostheses may help restore symmetry and support. These prostheses are available in a variety of forms, sizes, and materials to accommodate individual tastes and demands.

In addition to changes in look, you may have limits in your range of motion or strength, especially if lymph nodes were removed during surgery. Physical therapy and mild exercises advised by your doctor may help you gain mobility and avoid stiffness. Start cautiously and progressively raise your exercise levels as your body permits.

Psychological And Emotional Impact

The psychological and emotional consequences of mastectomy may be significant and diverse. Many people feel a variety of emotions after the operation, including sadness, fear, wrath, and worry. These sentiments are completely natural and might change in severity over time. It is important to allow oneself the freedom to experience and process these feelings without judgment.

Body image issues are also frequent after mastectomy. Adapting to changes in appearance and embracing a new physical reality might take time. It is common to be self-conscious or uneasy about your physique, particularly in personal or social situations. However, physical appearance alone does not determine beauty or value. Finding methods to recognize and celebrate your body's resiliency and strength may feel powerful.

Seeking assistance from friends, family, or a therapist may be quite beneficial at this time. Connecting with people who have had similar situations may give validation, understanding, and helpful coping strategies. Many hospitals and cancer support organizations provide support groups for those who have breast cancer or have had a mastectomy. These organizations may provide consolation and support as you face the difficulties of life after mastectomy.

Support Networks And Resources

Building a solid support network is critical for navigating life after a mastectomy. Surround yourself with individuals who support and encourage you, whether they be friends, family, or other survivors. Don't be afraid to rely on your support system for emotional support, practical help, or just company during tough times.

In addition to personal support networks, a variety of services and organizations may provide useful help and information. Cancer support groups like the American Cancer Society, Susan G. Komen, and Living Beyond Breast Cancer provide educational materials, online forums, helplines, and other resources for those impacted by breast cancer and mastectomy.

Your healthcare staff may also be a great source of information and advice. Please do not hesitate to ask questions or seek clarification on any part of your recovery or continuing treatment. Your medical team is there to help you and provide the information and resources you need to succeed.

Regaining Confidence And Embracing Your Body Image

Regaining confidence and adopting a good body image after mastectomy is a highly personal process that requires patience and self-compassion. Be patient with yourself and give yourself time to mourn, recover, and reclaim your sense of self-worth.

Finding activities or interests that make you happy and fulfilled might help you gain confidence and self-esteem. Whether it's painting, gardening, yoga, or volunteering, doing things that feed your soul and give you a sense of purpose may feel powerful.

Experimenting with different attire, haircuts, and cosmetics may be a fun way to express yourself and improve your self-esteem.

Many people discover that embracing their sense of style and originality makes them feel more confident and comfortable in their bodies.

Above all, realize that genuine beauty comes from inside. Accept your scars as symbols of strength and tenacity, and appreciate what your body has endured. You are more than your physical look, and your value is incalculable. With time, tolerance, and self-love, you can regain your confidence and face life after mastectomy with bravery and grace.

CHAPTER 10
Moving Forward

Follow-Up Care And Monitoring

Follow-up care and surveillance following a mastectomy are critical components of the healing process, maintaining the patient's health and detecting any possible problems early. The frequency and kind of follow-up care will be determined by the individual's medical history, cancer treatment details, and guidance from their healthcare team. Follow-up treatment usually involves frequent physical exams, mammography, and maybe other imaging tests.

Regular Physical Examinations

Regular physical exams by your healthcare practitioner are required. These check-ups enable physicians to evaluate your recovery, examine the surgery site for evidence of problems, and look for signs of recurrence or metastases. During these sessions, your doctor will also assess your general health, address any side effects or symptoms you may be experiencing, and provide advice on how to manage them.

Imaging Tests

Regular mammograms of the residual breast (if applicable) are recommended for patients who have had a mastectomy. Even if both breasts have been removed, imaging tests such as ultrasounds, MRIs, or bone scans may be needed depending on your unique risk factors. These tests aid in the early diagnosis of any recurrences or new malignancies, allowing for rapid treatment.

Self-Examination And Awareness

Patients should also do frequent self-examination and be mindful of changes in their bodies. Although self-exams on the excised breast are no longer possible, it is critical to monitor the surgical site and any leftover breast tissue. Report any new lumps, swelling, or strange symptoms to your doctor right away.

Reconstructive Surgery Follow-Up

If reconstructive surgery was part of your treatment plan, you should schedule follow-up appointments with your plastic surgeon. These meetings ensure that the reconstruction is healing well and that no problems arise, such as infections or implant concerns. Your surgeon will also look for symptoms of capsular contracture, which is scar tissue that forms around an implant.

Healthy Lifestyle Choices After Mastectomy

Adopting a healthy lifestyle after a mastectomy is critical for general well-being and lowering the chance of cancer reoccurrence.

This includes a balanced diet, frequent physical exercise, mental health treatment, and avoiding identified risk factors.

Balanced Nutrition

A diet rich in fruits, vegetables, whole grains, lean meats, and healthy fats promotes general health and immunological function. Limit your intake of processed meals, sugary beverages, and red meats, since they may all lead to inflammation and other health problems. A nutritionist can help you build a diet plan to your specific requirements and tastes, ensuring optimal nutritional consumption.

Regular Physical Activity

Exercise is helpful to both physical and mental well-being. It promotes a healthy weight, decreases stress, and enhances mood. Post-mastectomy, it is critical to gradually restore physical activity, beginning with mild workouts and progressively increasing intensity as tolerated. Walking, swimming, and yoga are all excellent exercise options. Before starting any new fitness plan, talk with your healthcare professional to confirm that it is safe and suitable.

Mental Health Care

A mastectomy may have a profound emotional effect, and dealing with mental health is an important part of the rehabilitation process. Support groups, therapy, and counseling may all give valuable emotional support. Mindfulness methods like meditation and deep breathing exercises may also help you manage stress and anxiety. Building a solid network of friends, family, and healthcare professionals is critical for emotional well-being.

Avoiding Risk Factors

A healthy lifestyle also includes avoiding recognized cancer risk factors. This involves giving up smoking, limiting alcohol use, and reducing exposure to environmental contaminants. Regular check-ups and screenings, along with a healthy lifestyle, may considerably minimize the likelihood of recurrence.

Advocacy And Awareness Efforts

Advocacy and awareness initiatives are critical to advancing breast cancer research, enhancing patient treatment, and supporting individuals impacted by the illness. Advocacy may be inspiring and give a chance to have a significant effect.

Participating In Advocacy Groups

Joining local or national breast cancer advocacy organizations enables people to help raise awareness and influence legislative changes. These groups often participate in fundraising, awareness events, and campaigning for research funding. Participation in these organizations may foster a feeling of belonging and purpose.

Sharing Personal Stories

Sharing your unique breast cancer journey might inspire and educate others. Personal tales, whether shared via speaking engagements, publishing articles or blog entries, or engaging in media campaigns, assist in humanizing the illness and highlighting the struggles and victories that survivors confront. These experiences might also provide hope and inspiration to people who are presently receiving therapy.

Raising Awareness

Raising awareness of breast cancer is critical for early identification and prevention. This might include planning or taking part in activities like breast cancer marches, awareness campaigns, and educational seminars. Social media platforms are an effective tool for raising awareness and sharing information with a large audience.

Supporting Research

Advocating for and funding breast cancer research is critical to developing novel therapies and strengthening current ones. This might involve taking part in clinical trials, giving to research organizations, and advocating for more research funding. Staying up to date on the newest scientific breakthroughs and sharing that knowledge with your community may help progress the battle against breast cancer.

Empowering Others With Personal Experience

Sharing personal experiences and offering support to others can be very powerful for both the giver and the recipient. By sharing your experience, you may provide hope, encouragement, and practical assistance to those facing similar issues.

Mentoring And Peer Support

Mentoring newly diagnosed patients may provide essential support and encouragement. Sharing your perspectives, coping tactics, and experiences might make others feel less alone and more powerful as they confront treatment and recovery. Many organizations provide peer support programs that link breast cancer survivors to others who are presently receiving treatment.

Educational Workshops & Seminars

Leading or participating in educational workshops and seminars enables you to share your expertise and experiences with a larger group. These events may include subjects such as dealing with a mastectomy, managing side effects, and navigating the healthcare system. Providing practical knowledge and tools might make people feel more prepared and educated.

Creative Expression

Writing, painting, and music are all effective ways to express and process your experiences. Sharing your creative work has the power to inspire and encourage others while also giving a unique and personal viewpoint on the breast cancer experience. Many survivors discover that artistic expression allows them to make sense of their experiences and find purpose in their path.

By actively participating in these activities, you not only benefit the larger community but also gain strength and resilience in your personal experience. Empowering people via your own story may be a satisfying component of moving on after a mastectomy.

Conclusion

To summarize, comprehending mastectomy entails acknowledging its varied character, from physical and emotional consequences to lifestyle adjustments and post-surgery care. A mastectomy is a surgical surgery that removes one or both breasts. It is generally used to cure or prevent breast cancer. The choice to have a mastectomy is very personal and may be impacted by a variety of variables such as genetic predisposition, cancer stage, and personal health concerns.

The road through mastectomy starts with understanding the many options: complete mastectomy, modified radical mastectomy, skin-sparing mastectomy, and nipple-sparing mastectomy. Each variety has unique indications, benefits, and hazards. A complete mastectomy, for example, removes all of the breast tissue while leaving the muscles below intact, but a modified radical mastectomy removes lymph nodes, which might be critical for staging cancer and deciding subsequent therapy.

Following surgery, patients confront a variety of physical and mental obstacles. Physical rehabilitation includes dealing with pain, surgery drains, and concerns like lymphedema, which is swelling caused by lymph fluid buildup. Physical therapy may be used throughout rehabilitation to help patients recover mobility and strength. Emotional healing is as important, since patients may endure emotions of loss, changes in body image, and the need for psychiatric care. Support groups, therapy, and open contact with loved ones may be quite beneficial for emotional rehabilitation.

Many people choose reconstructive surgery, which allows them to restore the contour and symmetry of their breasts. This may be done at the same time as the mastectomy or later. Implants and autologous tissue repair are two options for reconstruction, each with its own set of advantages and disadvantages. The decision to undergo reconstruction is very personal and should be decided in conjunction with healthcare specialists based on the patient's choices, health situation, and treatment objectives.

Advances in surgical procedures, anesthetic, and postoperative care have dramatically improved mastectomy patients' results and recovery experiences. Enhanced recovery after surgery (ERAS) procedures and less invasive treatments help to shorten hospital stays and accelerate recovery timeframes.

Finally, a thorough knowledge of mastectomy is essential for patients, caregivers, and healthcare practitioners. It enables patients to make more informed choices, creates a supportive atmosphere, and improves overall care quality. Taking a comprehensive approach to mastectomy rehabilitation that addresses both the physical and emotional components may dramatically enhance patients' long-term results and quality of life.

THE END